Mitochondrial Structure and Function

The Role of mitochondria in cellular processes.

Douglas Randall

Disclaimer

This book's content is intended solely for educational purposes and should not be used as medical advice. It should not be used for diagnosis or to take the place of professional medical monitoring. Before utilizing any of the information offered, it is advised that you discuss any medical issue with a healthcare professional.

The publisher and the author disclaim any responsibility for any harm purportedly caused by anything included in this book.

Content

Introduction

Overview of Mitochondria

A crucial organelle present in the cells of the majority of eukaryotes, including plants, animals, and fungi, is the mitochondrion. It is essential for the synthesis of cellular energy as well as several other cellular functions. This is a quick synopsis of the mitochondrial introduction:

Understanding and Organization: In the voluntary muscles of insects, Albert von Kölliker made the initial discovery of the mitochondrion in 1857. Its structure is double-membraned, with inner and outer membranes that produce what are known as cristae, or folds, in the inner membrane. The function of the organelle depends on several structures.

Energy Production: Aerobic respiration, the process by which mitochondria make adenosine triphosphate (ATP), the cellular energy currency, is the primary function of mitochondria. This is the main source of chemical energy for the cell and takes place in the inner mitochondrial membrane.

Mitochondrial DNA: Different from the nuclear DNA of the cell, mitochondria have their own little chromosomes and DNA. Mutations in mitochondrial DNA can result in a variety of illnesses. Generally, mitochondria and their DNA are inherited maternally.

Input into Cellular Mechanisms: Apart from generating energy, mitochondria are engaged in an extensive array of cellular functions, such as maintaining calcium balance, initiating cell death, and controlling the innate immune response.

Additionally, they are essential for eukaryotic cells' ability to produce metabolic energy.

Importance in Health and Disease: Mitochondria are essential for proper cellular operation and have been linked to a number of illnesses, such as cancer, metabolic diseases, and neurodegenerative disorders. Progress in these fields requires an understanding of their composition and operation.

The foundation for a more thorough examination of the composition and operation of mitochondria, as well as their vital role in biological functions and human health, is laid forth in this introduction.

Historical Perspective

Over numerous decades of scientific research, the historical perspective on mitochondrial structure and function has been intriguing. Known as the "powerhouses" of the cell, mitochondria are essential to many different cellular functions, and research on them has changed throughout the years. Since its inception in the pre-molecular era, mitochondrial medicine has progressed into the molecular age, which has seen notable conceptual and technological advancements. Numerous studies have been conducted on the function of mitochondria in oxidative phosphorylation, cellular bioenergetics, and the relationship between these processes and aging and illness. The dynamic nature of mitochondria, their role in the synthesis of cellular energy, and their influence on a range of physiological and pathological processes have all been made clear by research into their structure and function. The historical viewpoint on mitochondrial research sheds light on how our knowledge of these vital cellular organelles has evolved and how important they are to human health and disease.

Mitochondria play a variety of roles in cellular functions, including energy production, cell division, growth, and death. The dynamic, intricately structured organelles known as mitochondria, which have inner and outer membranes, are essential for preserving cellular equilibrium. Research on their role in age- and metabolic-related illnesses, as well as their effects on disease, inheritance, and cell viability, has been continuing. The importance of organelle morphology in defining their function and their role in various physiological and pathological processes has been highlighted by the research on mitochondrial structure and function.

The historical viewpoint on mitochondrial research sheds light on how our knowledge of these vital cellular organelles has evolved and how important they are to human health and disease. The dynamic nature of mitochondria, their role in the synthesis of cellular energy, and their influence on a range of physiological and pathological processes have all been made clear by research into their structure and function. Extensive research has been conducted on the role of mitochondria in oxidative phosphorylation, cellular bioenergetics, and their implications for aging and disease. Notable conceptual and technological advancements have marked the shift from the pre-molecular era to the molecular era of mitochondrial medicine.

Significance in Cellular Processes

Known as the "powerhouses" of the cell, mitochondria are essential to many different cellular functions, and research on them has changed throughout the years. The pre-molecular era provides the historical context for understanding mitochondrial structure and function. Since then, the molecular era—characterized by substantial conceptual and technological advancements—has been added to the historical viewpoint. Numerous studies have been conducted on the function of mitochondria in oxidative phosphorylation, cellular bioenergetics, and the relationship between these processes and aging and illness. The dynamic nature of mitochondria, their role in the synthesis of cellular energy, and their influence on a range of physiological and pathological processes have all been made clear by research into their structure and function.

The dynamic, intricately structured organelles known as mitochondria, which have inner and outer membranes, are essential for preserving cellular equilibrium. Research on their role in age- and metabolic-related illnesses, as well as their effects on disease, inheritance, and cell viability, has been continuing. The importance of organelle morphology in defining their function and their role in various physiological and pathological processes has been highlighted by the research on mitochondrial structure and function.

The historical viewpoint on mitochondrial research sheds light on how our knowledge of these vital cellular organelles has evolved and how important they are to human health and disease. The dynamic nature of mitochondria, their role in the synthesis of cellular energy, and their influence on a range of physiological and pathological processes have all been made clear by research into their structure and function. Extensive research has been conducted on the role of mitochondria in oxidative phosphorylation, cellular bioenergetics, and their implications for aging and disease. Notable conceptual and technological advancements have marked the shift from the pre-molecular era to the molecular era of mitochondrial medicine.

Chapter One

Mitochondrial Structure

Nearly all eukaryotic cells have mitochondria, which are organelles that carry out the process of oxidative phosphorylation to produce ATP, or energy. Their structure is double-membrane, with an inner and outer membrane divided by an intermembrane gap. The surface area available for ATP synthesis is increased by the inner membrane's many folds, or cristae. Among the cytoplasmic organelles, mitochondria are special because they have their own genome, which codes for tRNAs, rRNAs, and a few mitochondrial proteins. On free cytosolic ribosomes, the majority of mitochondrial proteins are translated and imported into the organelle. Other functions of mitochondria include the transmission of signals from cells to trigger programmed cell death, or apoptosis. In addition to age- and metabolic-related illnesses, extremely complex secondary diseases, including cancer, neurological disorders, heart disease, and stroke, are also linked to mitochondrial malfunction.

Outer and Inner Membrane

As stated earlier, Nearly all eukaryotic cells have mitochondria, which are organelles that carry out the process of oxidative phosphorylation to produce ATP, or energy. Their structure is double-membrane, with an inner and outer membrane divided by an intermembrane gap. The protein-to-phospholipid ratio of the outer mitochondrial membrane is roughly 1:1 by weight, and it is between 60 and 75 angstroms (Å) thick. It has a high concentration of porins, integral membrane proteins that create channels that permit the free flow of molecules smaller than roughly 6,000 daltons. In terms of ions, the intermembrane space and cytosol have similar compositions. The inner mitochondrial membrane, on the other hand, creates compartments by isolating the matrix from the cytosolic environment and is far less permeable to ions and small molecules than the outer membrane.

The inner mitochondrial membrane is highly folded and divided, with many membrane insertions known as cristae that are divided from the inner border membrane by crista junctions when positioned against the outer membrane. When compared to an inner membrane that is smooth, cristae greatly enhance the membrane's overall surface area. The outer mitochondrial membrane has a 50:50 protein-to-lipid ratio, but the inner membrane has an 80:20 ratio. Compared to the outer membrane, the inner membrane is substantially less permeable to ions and small molecules and is freely permeable to oxygen, carbon dioxide, and water alone.

The synthesis of ATP and electron transport chain processes occur within the inner mitochondrial membrane. Its integrity affects both the health and malfunction of mitochondria. Age- and metabolic-related illnesses, as well as extremely complex secondary diseases like cancer, neurological problems, heart disease, or stroke, are all linked to mitochondrial dysfunction.

Cristae and Matrix

The active organelles, known as mitochondria, are essential to the synthesis of energy in cells. Their double-membrane system, which consists of an outer and an inner membrane, gives them a distinct structure. The inner membrane creates what are known as cristae, which greatly expand the surface area available for the synthesis of ATP, the cell's energy currency. The majority of the electron transport chain complexes and ATP synthase are located in the cristae, which serve as the primary location for biological energy conversion. This makes it possible to produce ATP effectively, which is necessary for a number of cellular functions.

The inner mitochondrial membrane encloses the matrix, which is the innermost compartment of the mitochondrion. Numerous metabolic activities, including the citric acid cycle and fatty acid production, as well as enzymes involved in biosynthesis, are found there. The mitochondrial ribosomes, which are in charge of converting the mitochondrial genome into proteins, are also housed in the matrix. These proteins are involved in a number of cellular activities and are necessary for the mitochondria to operate.

Proper functioning of the mitochondria depends on the integrity of the cristae and matrix. Mitochondrial dysfunction, which is linked to a variety of illnesses such as metabolic disorders, neurodegenerative diseases, and cardiovascular ailments, can result from disruption of these structures. Thus, in order to comprehend the role of mitochondria in cellular activities and their consequences for health and disease, one must have a thorough understanding of the structure and function of the cristae and matrix.

Under physiological settings, the architecture and functions of the mitochondrial cristae are continuously undergoing cycles of membrane remodeling, which are governed by different protein and lipid compositions. Among the important participants in the morphological structuration of cristae are the protein OPA1, the dimers of ATP synthase, and the mitochondrial contact site and cristae organizing system (MICOS) system. Additionally, the structure and function of mitochondria are significantly influenced by the lipid composition, especially phosphatidylethanolamine (PE), which also serves to compensate for cardiolipin (CL) shortages and affect ATP synthesis.

In conclusion, the cristae and matrix are essential elements of mitochondrial structure and function, having a major impact on the metabolism and synthesis of cellular energy. Determining the wider consequences of mitochondrial function in health and disease requires an understanding of the mechanisms that control their integrity and organization.

Electron Microscopy Studies

The ultrastructure of mitochondria has been extensively studied thanks to electron microscopy, which has produced high-resolution images that have greatly advanced our knowledge of their structure and function. Although electron microscopy and electron tomography provide the finest resolution currently available to examine mitochondrial ultrastructure, light microscopy is still useful for observing mitochondrial function within cells.

The inner mitochondrial membrane is a major subject of electron microscopy research because of its many folds, or cristae. These cristae are essential for controlling the activity of the enzymes involved in the processes that produce reactive oxygen species and energy conversion. Furthermore, electron microscopy has been utilized to see the mitochondrial matrix, which at current resolution levels appears to be unstructured. Because of this, scientists have been able to examine how the mitochondrial matrix is organized and how it functions in different metabolic processes.

Studies using electron microscopy have also been crucial in describing the morphological alterations in mitochondria linked to various cellular states. For example, in cells going through certain physiological processes, vesicular morphology and swelling in the mitochondria have been seen, and electron microscopy has been essential in describing these morphological changes.

To sum up, the use of electron microscopy has proven to be indispensable in the investigation of mitochondrial structure and function. It has yielded an unparalleled understanding of the mitochondrial ultrastructure, including the arrangement of cristae and the mitochondrial matrix. These findings have ramifications for a range of physiological and pathological disorders and have greatly expanded our understanding of the role of mitochondria in cellular activities.

Chapter Two

Molecular Composition of Mitochondria

The intricate molecular makeup of mitochondria, which is necessary for their proper operation, makes them distinct organelles. The molecular makeup of mitochondria consists of minerals, granules, proteins, lipids, RNA, and DNA. The composition of the mitochondria is composed of 60–70% proteins, 25–35% lipids, 5–7% RNA, and trace amounts of DNA. There are also trace amounts of granules and minerals.

Encoding 37 genes, the mitochondrial genome is a circular, 16-kilobases double-stranded DNA molecule. These genes comprise 2 for rRNA, 22 for mitochondrial tRNA, and 13 for components of respiratory complexes I, III, IV, and V. The DNA of a single mitochondrion can be found in two to 10 copies.

The functional barrier that prevents tiny molecules from passing through between the cytosol and the matrix is the inner mitochondrial membrane. It has an abnormally high proportion (more than 70%) of proteins involved in the transfer of metabolites (including pyruvate and fatty acids) between the mitochondria and the cytoplasm. These proteins are also involved in oxidative phosphorylation. Because proteins called porins produce channels that allow molecules smaller than approximately 6,000 daltons to freely diffuse, the outer mitochondrial membrane is permeable to tiny molecules. Regarding ions, the intermembrane space's composition is comparable to that of the cytosol.

Any alteration to the molecular makeup of mitochondria can result in both cellular harm and dysfunction of the organelles. Gaining knowledge about the molecular makeup of mitochondria is crucial to comprehending their function in cellular activities and the consequences of these processes for both health and sickness.

Proteins and Lipids

Lipids and proteins are crucial for the structure and operation of the mitochondria. Lipids comprise 25–35% of the mitochondrial makeup, while proteins make up 60–70% of it. Fatty acids, glycerophospholipids, glycerolipids, sphingolipids, and prenols are among the molecules that make up mitochondria. The mitochondrial membrane's lipid composition is tailored to the organelle's structural arrangements and appropriate functions.

An exceptionally high proportion (more than 70%) of the proteins involved in oxidative phosphorylation and the movement of metabolites (such as pyruvate and fatty acids) between the cytosol and mitochondria are found in the inner mitochondrial membrane. Because proteins known as porins exist and provide channels that permit the free transport of molecules smaller than roughly 6,000 daltons, the outer mitochondrial membrane is open to small molecules.

Lipids are essential for the synthesis of energy, the integrity of the mitochondrial membrane, and signaling. Precursor lipids for mitochondrial lipid synthesis and other lipids are carried from other organelles, primarily the endoplasmic reticulum (ER), within the organelle. For optimal mitochondrial function, the composition, production, and import of mitochondrial lipids, as well as the regulation of these processes, are necessary.

Any alteration to the molecular makeup of mitochondria can result in both cellular harm and dysfunction of the organelles. Gaining knowledge about the molecular makeup of mitochondria is crucial to comprehending their function in cellular activities and the consequences of these processes for both health and sickness. Any alteration to the optimal lipid and protein composition of the mitochondrial membranes can result in mitochondrial malfunction and cellular damage, as well as improper organelle activities and structural arrangements.

Mitochondrial DNA (mtDNA)

The distinctive genetic material known as mitochondrial DNA (mtDNA) is located inside the mitochondria, which are the energy-producing organelles of eukaryotic cells. In contrast to nuclear DNA, which is found in the nucleus of the cell, mtDNA is a tiny, circular, double-stranded DNA molecule that makes up a small portion of all DNA in cells in humans. It consists of roughly 16,500 base pairs. It has 37 genes in total, all of which are necessary for regular mitochondrial activity. Thirteen of these genes encode the enzymes needed for oxidative phosphorylation, which produces adenosine triphosphate (ATP), the primary energy source for cells, by combining oxygen and simple carbohydrates. The remaining genes code for the production of substances known as ribosomal RNA (rRNA) and transfer RNA (tRNA).

Nuclear DNA is not the same as mtDNA due to its distinguishing features, such as its circular structure and absence of introns. Compared to nuclear DNA, it is inherited from the mother, is maternally inherited, and is more prone to mutation. Mutations in mtDNA can result in mitochondrial disorders, which can impact the body's systems, especially the neurological system and muscles, which have high energy requirements.

Understanding the function of mitochondria in cellular activities and the implications for health and disease requires an understanding of mtDNA. It has been useful in population genetics, maternal lineage tracking, and comprehending the genetic underpinnings of mitochondrial disorders. Furthermore, the special properties of mtDNA—such as its rapid rate of mutation and maternal inheritance—make it an invaluable resource for research on populations and evolution.

In conclusion, mtDNA encodes vital proteins and RNAs involved in energy production and cellular functions, making it a key part of mitochondrial structure and function. Because of its special qualities, it is a useful tool for studying population genetics, human evolution, and the genetics of mitochondrial disorders.

RNA and Protein Synthesis

A vital process called mitochondrial protein synthesis uses oxidative phosphorylation to produce the proteins needed for the synthesis of ATP. The mitochondrial ribosome, also known as the mitoribosome, facilitates this process, which takes place in the mitochondrial matrix. Different from the 80S ribosomes found in the cytoplasm of eukaryotes and the 70S ribosomes found in prokaryotes, the mitoribosome is a non-canonical ribosome.

<u>The production of mitochondrial proteins in mammals occurs in multiple steps</u>:

1. Transcription of nuclear genes: Messenger RNAs (mRNAs) are the first transcripts that are used to code for mitochondrial proteins in nuclear genes.

2. Mitochondrial protein production in the cytoplasm: The cytosolic ribosomes manufacture the nuclear-encoded proteins, which are then directed into the mitochondria and transported into the matrix.

3. Import of mitochondrial proteins: Several routes and large molecular machinery are involved in the import of mitochondrial proteins that are made in the cytoplasm. Translation of mRNAs initiates the targeting of some, but not all, cytoplasmically produced mitochondrial proteins.

4. Mt-mRNA translation: The constructed mitoribosome translates the mt-mRNAs, producing proteins that are quickly integrated into their appropriate sites and inserted into the inner mitochondrial membrane (IMM).

5. RNA processing: The poly(A) tail helps all light-strand protein-encoding RNAs mature, producing two dicistronic and nine monocistronic mt-mRNA species.

All animals require mitochondrial protein synthesis because it produces critical elements of oxidative phosphorylation complexes. Numerous mitochondrial components, such as initiation factors, elongation factors, release factors, and ribosome recycling factors, are involved in this intricate process. Gaining knowledge about the molecular aspects of this process is essential to comprehending the function of mitochondria in cellular activities and the implications of their functions in health and sickness.

Chapter Three

Bioenergetics and Oxidative Phosphorylation

In particular, through the process of oxidative phosphorylation, which is essential for the synthesis of ATP, the cell's main energy source, mitochondria play a crucial role in cellular bioenergetics. Proton pumping and a number of redox processes are involved in this process, which takes place in the inner mitochondrial membrane. The following are some important details about oxidative phosphorylation and bioenergetics in the structure and function of mitochondria:

1. Oxidative Phosphorylation: This metabolic process produces ATP by transferring electrons from NADH and FADH2 to oxygen. The inner mitochondrial membrane contains the electron transport chain (ETC), which is essential to oxidative phosphorylation. It is made up of ATP

synthase (complex V) and four protein complexes (I–IV), which combine to produce ATP.

2. Proton Pumping and Electrochemical Gradient: Protons are pumped across the inner mitochondrial membrane by electrons traveling via the electron transport chain (ETC), resulting in an electrochemical gradient. The ATP synthase enzyme is propelled to synthesize ATP by this gradient, which is a type of potential energy known as chemiosmosis.

3. Production of Reactive Oxygen Species (ROS): Although the ETC is necessary for the synthesis of ATP, it can also result in the secondary byproduct of reactive oxygen species (ROS). If ROS are not appropriately controlled, they can harm cellular structures and components of the mitochondria.

4. Bioenergetics and Mitochondrial Dynamics: The bioenergetic condition of

mitochondria is closely related to both their structure and dynamics. Certain proteins drive processes like fusion and fission, which aid in preserving mitochondrial function and adapting to variations in energy requirements.

5. Role in Disease and Ageing: A number of illnesses, as well as the aging process, have been related to mitochondrial malfunction and decreased bioenergetics. Bioenergetic balance and oxidative phosphorylation problems can have profound effects on the health and functionality of cells.

In conclusion, oxidative phosphorylation and other aspects of mitochondrial bioenergetics are critical for cellular energy balance and ATP synthesis. Determining the function of mitochondria in cellular activities and their consequences in health and disease requires an understanding of the complex mechanisms underlying mitochondrial bioenergetics.

ATP Production

The principal energy source of the cell, ATP, is produced mostly by mitochondria through a process known as oxidative phosphorylation. The mitochondrial ATP synthase, a crucial enzyme that uses the energy from the proton electrochemical gradient to synthesize ATP from ADP and inorganic phosphate, is involved in this process, which takes place in the inner mitochondrial membrane.

The electron transport chain (ETC) makes it easier for electrons to move from NADH and FADH2 to oxygen during oxidative phosphorylation. An electrochemical gradient is produced by pumping protons across the inner mitochondrial membrane using the energy released by this electron transport. The ATP synthase then uses the proton motive force created by this gradient to convert ADP and inorganic phosphate into ATP.

Numerous biological functions, such as protein synthesis, muscular contraction, and membrane potential maintenance, depend on the ATP synthase found in the mitochondria to provide energy. In eukaryotic cells, mitochondria are the primary source of ATP, and their capacity to produce ATP is essential for maintaining essential cellular processes.

To summarize, the energy currency that powers vital biological functions is produced by the mitochondrial ATP synthase through oxidative phosphorylation. To fully comprehend the role of mitochondria in cellular processes and the consequences for health and disease, it is imperative to get an understanding of the structure and function of ATP synthase as well as the process of oxidative phosphorylation.

Electron Transport Chain

A crucial element of mitochondrial structure and function, the electron transport chain

(ETC) is essential to cellular bioenergetics. It is the principal location of oxidative phosphorylation, which produces ATP, the major energy unit of the cell. A number of chemical compounds and protein complexes embedded in the inner mitochondrial membrane make up the ETC. An electrochemical gradient is produced when protons are pumped across the inner mitochondrial membrane by the energy released by electrons as they pass through the ETC. This gradient, which is a type of potential energy, is what propels ATP synthase's production of ATP—a process called chemiosmosis.

Together with other electron carriers, the four large protein complexes designated I through IV make up the ETC. These complexes are located in the inner mitochondrial membrane of eukaryotes. In order to produce ATP, the electrons from NADH or FADH2 must travel to oxygen, the terminal electron acceptor, with the help of the electron transport chain (ETC). The preservation of cellular energy balance and the regeneration of electron carriers depend on this process.

Reactive oxygen species (ROS), which can harm cellular components and cause signaling, are also produced in large quantities by the ETC. As a natural byproduct of the ETC, ROS formation must be controlled in order to preserve cellular homeostasis.

In conclusion, the electron transport chain is an essential part of the structure and operation of the mitochondria and is crucial to the synthesis of ATP and cellular bioenergetics. To fully comprehend the function of mitochondria in cellular processes and the consequences for health and disease, one must have a thorough understanding of the mechanisms and regulation of the ETC.

Oxidative Phosphorylation Process

A crucial step in the formation and operation of mitochondria, oxidative phosphorylation is essential to cellular bioenergetics. It is the principal process by which ATP, the principal energy unit of the cell, is produced. The electron transport chain (ETC) and ATP synthase are involved in this process, which takes place in the inner mitochondrial membrane.

The general mechanism of oxidative phosphorylation is chemiosmotic coupling, whereby the mitochondrial electron transport chain catalyzes the oxidation of respiratory substrates by oxygen, which results in the extrusion of protons across the inner membrane of the mitochondria. Protons are driven back into the mitochondrial matrix by the proton-motive force created by this proton pumping, and ATP synthase uses this energy to synthesize ATP.

A collection of chemical compounds and protein complexes embedded in the inner mitochondrial membrane make up the electron transport chain (ETC). An electrochemical gradient is produced when protons are pumped across the inner mitochondrial membrane by the energy released by electrons as they pass through the ETC. The ATP synthase enzyme is propelled to synthesize ATP by this gradient, which is a type of potential energy known as chemiosmosis.

In eukaryotic cells, oxidative phosphorylation is the main source of ATP due to its high efficiency in producing the molecule. It is necessary to sustain basic cellular processes like muscle contraction, protein synthesis, and membrane potential maintenance.

In conclusion, oxidative phosphorylation is an essential mechanism for the structure and operation of mitochondria, being crucial to the synthesis of ATP and the bioenergetics of cells. Gaining insight into the mechanics and control of oxidative phosphorylation is crucial in determining the function of mitochondria in cellular activities and the consequences they have for both health and illness.

Chapter Four

Mitochondrial Dynamics

The processes of fusion and fission that mitochondria go through inside particular cells are referred to as mitochondrial dynamics. Because of these processes, mitochondria develop a morphological spectrum with differing levels of elongation and fragmentation, which enables them to adapt to shifting cellular stressors and continue to function. Numerous cellular functions, including immunology, apoptosis, and mitochondrial quality control, depend on the balance between fusion and fission events in order to preserve the size, shape, and distribution of mitochondria.

<u>Important facets of the dynamics of mitochondria include</u>:

1. Fusion and Fission: The precise cycles of fusion and fission that mitochondria go through are necessary to preserve their size, distribution, and shape. Whereas fission events split mitochondria into smaller components, fusion events unite them.

2. Dynamin-related Proteins: Mitochondrial fusion is primarily regulated by the equilibrium amongst four dynamin-related proteins (Drp1, Mfn1/2, and Opa1). These proteins are engaged in many different cellular activities and are essential in controlling mitochondrial dynamics.

3. Mitochondrial Dynamics Proteins: These proteins have a role in controlling the size, shape, and dispersion of mitochondria. Under a number of circumstances, dysfunction of these proteins has been suggested as a potential disease mechanism.

4. ER-Actin Membranes: Post-translational changes of important proteins, lipid composition, and endoplasmic reticulum (ER)-actin membranes are some of the numerous regulatory layers that govern mitochondrial dynamics.

5. Physiological Functions and Disorders: Fission and fusion of mitochondria control a wide range of physiological processes and are implicated in a number of disorders. Numerous health problems have been connected to abnormalities in mitochondrial dynamics and mutations in the essential machinery components.

In conclusion, a variety of cellular activities as well as the preservation of mitochondrial size, shape, and distribution depend heavily on mitochondrial dynamics. Deciphering the function of mitochondria in cellular activities and their consequences for health and illness requires an understanding of the molecular mechanisms and regulation of mitochondrial dynamics.

Fission and Fusion

Fission and fusion are two fundamental processes known as mitochondrial dynamics that control the shape, location, and functionality of mitochondria in cells. These dynamic processes are strictly controlled and are essential for preserving cellular homeostasis and mitochondrial function. The following are some important details about fission and fusion in the structure and operation of mitochondria:

1. Fission: The process by which a single mitochondrion splits into two or more offspring organelles is known as mitochondrial fission. The regulation of mitochondrial size, distribution, and quality control is contingent upon this mechanism. A group of proteins control it: fission protein 1 (Fis1) and mitochondrial fission factor (Mff), which attract Drp1 to the outer

membrane of the mitochondria, and dynamin-related protein 1 (Drp1), which contracts and divides the mitochondrial membrane.

2. Merger: The merger of two distinct mitochondria into a single, networked organelle is known as mitochondrial fusion. This process is essential for maintaining a healthy population of mitochondria within the cell, supplementing the mitochondrial genome, and combining the contents of partially damaged mitochondria. Optic atrophy 1 (OPA1) mediates the fusing of the inner mitochondrial membrane, whereas mitofusin 1 and 2 (Mfn1 and Mfn2) are the GTPases in charge of the fusion of the outer mitochondrial membrane.

3. Participation in Cellular Illness and Health: The health of cells and the operation of mitochondria depend on the balance between fission and fusion. Numerous illnesses, including cancer, metabolic

diseases, and neurodegenerative disorders, have been related to the dysregulation of these systems. For instance, poor fusion can hamper energy generation and cellular homeostasis, whereas excessive fission might accumulate damaged mitochondria.

4. Regulation: A number of cellular processes, such as proteolytic processing, ubiquitylation, sumoylation, phosphorylation, and dephosphorylation, carefully control fission and fusion. In order to adapt to cellular and metabolic needs, stress, and damage, mitochondrial dynamics must be precisely regulated, which is ensured by several regulatory mechanisms.

To sum up, fission and fusion are essential processes for maintaining the morphology, distribution, and quality control of mitochondria, and they are vital to mitochondrial structure and function. Deciphering the function of mitochondria in cellular processes and their consequences for health and disease requires an understanding of the molecular mechanisms and regulation of these processes.

Mitochondrial Movement

One important component of mitochondrial dynamics is mitochondrial mobility, which is the movement and repositioning of these organelles inside cells. Ensuring appropriate mitochondrial function and preserving cellular homeostasis depend on this process. Motor proteins, cytoskeletal components, and regulatory factors work in concert to promote mitochondrial movement, which is essential for many cellular functions. The following are some essential details about mitochondrial mobility in relation to mitochondrial structure and function:

1. Intracellular Transport: Motor proteins like dynein and kinesin connect to mitochondria to facilitate movement within the cell along cytoskeletal components, mainly microtubules. Mitochondria can be

distributed to areas of the cell where energy needs are high, like the cell periphery or locations of active metabolism, thanks to this transport.

2. Control of Mitochondrial Distribution: To guarantee that these organelles are dispersed throughout the cell adequately, mitochondrial mobility is strictly controlled. Meeting the varying dynamic energy demands of distinct cellular areas and preserving cellular homeostasis depend on this regulation.

3. Input into Cellular Mechanisms: Numerous cellular functions, such as cell migration, division, and polarity maintenance, depend on mitochondrial mobility. Additionally, it is essential for supplying energy to particular subcellular areas, such as the leading edge of a migrating cell or the development cone of a growing neuron.

4. Implications in Health and Disease: A number of diseases, including metabolic and neurodegenerative disorders, have been related to dysregulation of mitochondrial movement. Comprehending the mechanisms that regulate the movement of mitochondria is crucial in order to decipher the function of mitochondria in cellular activities and their consequences in both health and illness.

To summarize, the migration of mitochondria is an essential activity in the construction and function of mitochondria, and it is crucial for preserving cellular homeostasis and satisfying the varying energy requirements of several cellular regions. Deciphering the function of mitochondria in cellular processes and their consequences for health and illness requires an understanding of the molecular mechanisms and regulation of mitochondrial mobility.

Quality Control and Turnover

The vital functions of mitochondrial quality management and turnover govern the health and functionality of mitochondria in cells. These procedures are essential for preserving the homeostasis of cells and guaranteeing healthy mitochondrial operation. The following are some salient features of mitochondrial turnover and quality control in relation to mitochondrial structure and function:

1. Control of Mitochondrial Quality: A group of evolutionary-conserved processes known as mitochondrial quality control (MQC) work to preserve the mitochondrial proteome in order to support the proper operation of the organelle and, consequently, the health of the cell [4]. These processes include the folding, degrading, and turnover of proteins in addition to the dynamics of the mitochondria, which control the shape and distribution of the mitochondria.

2. Mitochondrial Turnover: Autophagy and mitophagy are two essential processes for the selective elimination of malfunctioning mitochondria during mitochondrial turnover, which is a crucial component of quality control. This procedure is necessary to keep the cell's mitochondria in good health and to stop damaged organelles from building up.

3. Role in Cellular Activities: Cell division, migration, and the preservation of cellular polarity are only a few of the activities in which mitochondrial quality control and turnover are essential. Additionally, they are essential in supplying energy to particular subcellular areas, like the leading edge of a migrating cell or the development cone of a growing neuron.

4. Implications in Health and Disease: Cancer, metabolic disorders, neurodegenerative diseases, and other

diseases have all been related to dysregulation of mitochondrial quality control and turnover. Deciphering the function of mitochondria in cellular processes and their consequences in health and illness requires an understanding of the mechanisms governing mitochondrial quality control and turnover.

To sum up, the mechanisms of mitochondrial quality control and turnover are essential to the structure and function of mitochondria, and they are crucial in preserving cellular homeostasis and averting the buildup of damaged organelles. Deciphering the function of mitochondria in cellular processes and their consequences for health and disease requires an understanding of the molecular mechanisms and regulation of these processes.

Chapter Five

Mitochondrial Function in Cellular Processes

Numerous cellular functions, such as energy production, metabolism, and signaling, depend on mitochondrial activity. Through a process that takes place in the inner mitochondrial membrane called oxidative phosphorylation, mitochondria are in charge of producing ATP, the primary energy source of the cell. In addition, mitochondria are essential for the synthesis of amino acids and phospholipids, as well as for the control of apoptosis, calcium homeostasis, and the creation of heme and iron-sulfur clusters.

Numerous processes, such as turnover, quality control, and mitochondrial dynamics, carefully govern mitochondrial activity. Fission and fusion are two fundamental processes known as mitochondrial dynamics that control the shape, location, and functionality of mitochondria in cells. These dynamic processes are strictly controlled and are essential for preserving cellular homeostasis and mitochondrial health.

The vital functions of mitochondrial quality management and turnover govern the health and functionality of mitochondria in cells. These procedures are essential for preserving the homeostasis of cells and guaranteeing healthy mitochondrial operation. Protein folding, breakdown, and turnover, as well as mitochondrial dynamics, which govern mitochondrial morphology and distribution, are examples of mechanisms for controlling the quality of mitochondria.

Numerous diseases, including cancer, metabolic problems, and neurological diseases, have been related to dysregulation of mitochondrial activity. Deciphering the function of mitochondria in cellular activities and their consequences for health and illness requires an understanding of the mechanisms that control mitochondrial activity.

In conclusion, a variety of cellular functions, such as energy production, metabolism, and signaling, depend on mitochondrial activity. Essential processes that govern mitochondrial activity and guarantee appropriate cellular homeostasis include turnover, quality control, and mitochondrial dynamics. Understanding the function of mitochondria in cellular activities is crucial, as evidenced by the numerous diseases that have been associated with dysregulation of mitochondrial function.

Energy Metabolism

An essential part of eukaryotic cells' energy metabolism is played by mitochondria. They are in charge of the process known as oxidative phosphorylation, which takes place in the inner mitochondrial membrane and produces ATP, the main energy source for the cell. Three primary mechanisms are involved in mitochondrial energy metabolism in cells: oxidative phosphorylation, the TCA cycle, and glycolysis. Reduced flavin adenine dinucleotide, reduced nicotinamide adenine dinucleotide (NADH), and other energetic molecules are produced by glycolysis and the TCA cycle, and oxidative phosphorylation uses these materials to reduce O2 and release energy to synthesize ATP.

The regulation of multiple cellular activities, such as cell migration, division, and polarity maintenance, depends on mitochondrial function. Additionally, mitochondria are essential for supplying energy to particular subcellular areas, such as the leading edge of a migrating cell or the development cone of a growing neuron.

The complexity of mitochondrial metabolism extends well beyond bioenergetics. In order to maintain redox equilibrium, compartmentalize metabolites for energy production, produce biosynthetic precursors for macromolecules, and act as centers for metabolic waste management, all of these are accomplished by mitochondria. Numerous activities in cell biology are supported by mitochondrial metabolism, and a better comprehension of the contributions made by mitochondria to metabolism will clarify the role that these organelles play in cellular functioning.

In conclusion, mitochondrial activity is critical for eukaryotic cells' energy metabolism since it affects cellular bioenergetics and ATP synthesis. Additionally, mitochondria are essential for controlling a number of biological functions, such as cell migration, division, and polarity maintenance. Deciphering the function of mitochondria in cellular activities and the consequences for health and disease requires an understanding of the molecular mechanisms and regulation of mitochondrial function.

Calcium Homeostasis

Because calcium is involved in so many different biological activities, maintaining calcium homeostasis is an essential component of mitochondrial structure and function. Since the endoplasmic reticulum (ER) and mitochondria contain the majority of calcium, they are essential for controlling calcium levels throughout the cell. The maintenance of cellular health and the appropriate operation of numerous cellular activities depend on calcium homeostasis.

The precise mechanism that determines the mitochondria's ability to handle calcium governs the maintenance of mitochondrial calcium homeostasis. Cell survival and the control of aerobic metabolism depend on this process. The dynamics, function, and metabolism of mitochondria are correlated with their calcium levels, and mitochondria are implicated in cellular microdomains that control essential cellular processes.

<u>Important elements of calcium homeostasis in mitochondria include:</u>

1. Calcium Transport: The uptake of calcium into the mitochondrial matrix is carried out by specific calcium transport systems found in mitochondria, such as the mitochondrial calcium uniporter (MCU). Calcium homeostasis is facilitated by a number of other mechanisms, including the mitochondrial permeability transition pore (mPTP).

2. Calcium Buffering: The ability of mitochondria to buffer calcium contributes to the maintenance of intracellular calcium levels [2]. Proteins carry out this buffering, and other processes, like the buffer system,

that maintain calcium homeostasis are merely temporary and have little effect on the calcium concentration over the long run.

3. Calcium Signaling: Cell migration and other cellular functions are influenced by intracellular calcium signals, whose timing and amplitude are greatly influenced by mitochondria.

4. Calcium and ATP Synthesis: The generation of ATP, which is necessary for the synthesis of cellular energy, is aided by calcium in the mitochondria.

Cancer and neurological illnesses have both been related to dysregulation of mitochondrial calcium homeostasis. Deciphering the function of mitochondria in cellular processes and their consequences for health and illness requires an understanding of the molecular mechanisms and regulation of mitochondrial calcium homeostasis.

Apoptosis and Cell Signaling

Particularly through the mitochondrial pathway of apoptosis, mitochondria are essential for both cell signaling and apoptosis. The activation of caspases, which in turn causes cell death, is triggered by the release of apoptotic proteins, such as cytochrome c, from the mitochondrial intermembrane gap. One important step in this process is the permeabilization of the outer membrane of the mitochondria, which is controlled by a number of proteins and processes, such as the mitochondrial permeability transition pore (mPTP) and members of the Bcl-2 family.

Apoptosis via the mitochondrial route is a tightly controlled process that is necessary for removing unhealthy or undesired cells and preserving cellular homeostasis. This pathway's dysregulation has been connected to a number of illnesses, including cancer, and it is a major target for the creation of cutting-edge anti-cancer medications.

Apart from apoptosis, mitochondria also participate in other types of programmed cell death, like necroptosis. Furthermore, they are essential for controlling other cellular functions, such as cell division, growth, and cell cycle regulation. Biogenesis and autophagy carefully control the dynamic character of mitochondria, including their location and form inside cells, maintaining a comparatively stable population of mitochondria.

In conclusion, mitochondria coordinate the synthesis of energy within cells and are essential to normal cellular function. They are essential for both apoptosis and cell signaling, especially via the mitochondrial apoptotic pathway. They also regulate a number of other cellular functions, such as cell division, growth, and cycle regulation. In the fields of cell biology and medicine, comprehending the complex role that mitochondrial function plays in cell

viability, illness, and inheritance is a crucial
subject of ongoing research.

Chapter Six

Mitochondria-Associated Diseases

The synthesis of phospholipids and other forms of energy production in eukaryotes is carried out by mitochondria, which are essential to regular cellular activity. They serve as both the gatekeepers of cell death and the maintenance of life. Numerous essential cellular activities, such as cell proliferation and differentiation, cell cycle regulation, and cell death, are facilitated by mitochondria. The location and form of mitochondria in cells are essential and strictly controlled by the processes of autophagy and biogenesis, which maintain a comparatively stable number of mitochondria. The problems associated with aging and metabolism are linked to mitochondrial malfunction. The significance of organelle morphology in determining function is highlighted by the modulation of mitochondrial morphology, which is linked to disease states and is influenced by the balance between fission and fusion events. Additional regulatory layers, including the ER-actin membranes, lipid composition, and post-translational changes of important proteins, govern the dynamics of mitochondria. Numerous physiological processes are regulated by mitochondrial fission and fusion, which also play a role in a number of illnesses. Numerous uncertainties remain, and our understanding of the complex role that mitochondrial activity plays in cell survival, illness, and inheritance is still developing. Because of their function in the synthesis of energy, mitochondria are frequently referred to as the "powerhouse of the cell." But throughout the past 30 years, mitochondria have also been identified as a signaling organelle engaged in a variety of activities, such as the formation of heme and iron-sulfur clusters, calcium homeostasis, and apoptosis. Cells use the process of dephosphorylating an ATP molecule to produce an ADP molecule as their primary energy source. The extremely active organelles known as mitochondria reconfigure their network to preserve their size and distribution. Depending on the physiological requirements of the cell, the balance between fission and fusion events modifies the morphology of the mitochondria. The Dynamin family of large GTPases comprises the constituents of the main machinery responsible for controlling mitochondrial dynamics. Numerous physiological processes are regulated by mitochondrial fission and fusion, which also play a role in a number of illnesses.

Mitochondrial Disorders

A class of hereditary and acquired ailments collectively referred to as mitochondrial diseases or disorders are brought on by malfunctioning mitochondria. These conditions can impact different body systems and organs, resulting in a broad spectrum of symptoms. Since mitochondria are the main locations for ATP synthesis, poor energy generation is frequently a defining feature of mitochondrial diseases. The signs and symptoms of illnesses related to the mitochondria might differ greatly because different tissues and organs demand different amounts of energy. Muscle weakness, neurological disorders, heart problems, and eye impairments are common symptoms. Moreover, a number of illnesses, including cancer, metabolic problems, and neurological diseases, have been connected to mitochondrial abnormalities. Understanding the molecular mechanisms and regulation of mitochondrial function is crucial for deciphering the role of mitochondria in cellular processes and their consequences in health and illness. Research on mitochondrial disorders is an active field.

Role in Age-Related Diseases

An important factor in aging and age-related disorders is mitochondria. A growing body of research indicates a causal connection between major age-related illnesses such as cancer, cardiovascular disease, and neurodegenerative disorders and mitochondrial dysfunction. A number of aging-related phenomena are linked to mitochondrial dysfunction, such as decreased activity of metabolic enzymes, oxidative phosphorylation impairment, elevated oxidative damage, deterioration in mitochondrial quality control, and modifications to the shape, dynamics, and biogenesis of mitochondria. Many studies have been conducted on the role of mitochondria in aging, and it has been shown that one of the main indicators of aging is mitochondrial malfunction. One of the main indicators of aging is mitochondrial dysfunction, which is related to the management of energy and metabolic balance. In order to design therapies to reduce age-related pathologies and enhance health outcomes, it is imperative to comprehend the multifaceted role that mitochondrial activity plays in aging and age-related disorders. This is an area of ongoing research.

Mitochondrial Dysfunction in Cancer

Numerous human diseases, such as gynecologic cancers, neurological disorders, cardiovascular diseases, and cancer, have been linked to mitochondrial malfunction. Cancer has been implicated in several conditions. Changes in both structure and function that can impact mitochondrial function are indicative of mitochondrial dysfunction in cancer. Aggression of the disease is correlated with the level of mitochondrial malfunction, emphasizing the mitochondrion as a critical target for diagnosis and treatment.

The metabolism of cancer cells depends heavily on mitochondria, and abnormalities in these organelles can affect the invasiveness, metastasis, and therapeutic responsiveness of cancer cells. Awareness of mitochondrial bioenergetics in cancer cells requires an awareness of mitochondrial malfunction, and comprehending mitochondrial function in cancer cells requires measuring mitochondrial parameters.

Numerous modifications to mitochondrial structure and function, such as changes to cristae shape, mitochondrial DNA integrity and quantity, bioenergetic capability, calcium retention, and membrane potential, are linked to mitochondrial dysfunction in cancer. These modifications may have an impact on mitochondrial activity and aid in the etiology of cancer.

To reduce cancer pathologies and enhance health outcomes, therapies to regulate mitochondrial dysfunction in cancer must be developed with a thorough understanding of the molecular pathways underlying the condition. Research on mitochondrial malfunction in cancer is ongoing and crucial to understanding the function of mitochondria in cellular activities and the consequences for health and disease.

Chapter Seven

Regulation of Mitochondrial Function

Numerous systems that guarantee appropriate cellular functions and preserve cellular homeostasis control mitochondrial function. These mechanisms encompass turnover, quality control, and mitochondrial dynamics. Fission and fusion are two fundamental processes known as mitochondrial dynamics that control the shape, location, and functionality of mitochondria in cells. These dynamic processes are strictly controlled and are essential for preserving cellular homeostasis and mitochondrial health.

The vital functions of mitochondrial quality management and turnover govern the health and functionality of mitochondria in cells. These procedures are essential for preserving the homeostasis of cells and guaranteeing healthy mitochondrial operation. Protein folding, degradation, and turnover, as well as mitochondrial dynamics, which govern mitochondrial morphology and distribution, are examples of methods for controlling the quality of mitochondria.

Numerous processes, such as turnover, quality control, and mitochondrial dynamics, carefully govern mitochondrial activity. Numerous diseases, including cancer, metabolic problems, and neurological diseases, have been related to dysregulation of mitochondrial activity. Deciphering the role of mitochondria in cellular processes and their consequences for health and disease requires an understanding of the molecular mechanisms and regulation of mitochondrial function.

In conclusion, a variety of mechanisms that guarantee appropriate cellular functions and preserve cellular homeostasis govern mitochondrial function. These mechanisms encompass turnover, quality control, and mitochondrial dynamics. Numerous diseases have been associated with dysregulation of mitochondrial function, underscoring the significance of comprehending the molecular mechanisms and regulation of mitochondrial function in cellular activities, as well as its consequences in both health and disease.

Nuclear-Mitochondrial Communication

The primary energy providers in a cell, mitochondria also serve as signaling hubs, facilitating direct and indirect interactions with other organelles. Nuclear DNA encodes most of the proteins found in mitochondria, even though it has its own circular genome. The nucleus, which has the ability to control mitochondrial function, receives signals from the mitochondria in response to modifications in cell physiology. Mito-nuclear communication is the term for this bidirectional connection that is necessary for coordinating different cellular processes and preserving cellular homeostasis. Through a multitude of processes, such as the synthesis and release of mitochondrial metabolites, the creation of reactive oxygen species (ROS), and the control of mitochondrial dynamics and quality control, mitochondria interact with the nucleus. Numerous cellular processes, including energy consumption, cell cycle regulation, and stress responses, are impacted by these signals because they have the ability to affect nuclear gene expression, chromatin structure, and epigenetic alterations. Research on how different substances, such as B vitamins, regulate mito-nuclear communication has become more significant because of its potential to understand and cure a wide range of human diseases, such as cancer, neurodegenerative diseases, and metabolic disorders. It is anticipated that research on mito-nuclear communication, an area that is dynamic and quickly developing, will provide significant new understandings of the function of mitochondria in cellular processes and how these functions relate to both health and sickness.

Mitochondrial Biogenesis

The process by which new mitochondria are created from pre-existing ones is known as mitochondrial biogenesis. Energy needs are met by this process, which entails the expansion and division of pre-existing mitochondria in response to environmental stressors and developmental cues. The nuclear and mitochondrial genomes must coordinate during this intricate, multi-step process of self-renewal. Nuclear DNA encodes most mitochondrial proteins, and the transcription, translation, regulation of mitochondrial dynamics, and quality control of mitochondrial DNA are all part of the process of mitochondrial biogenesis.

Many factors, including environmental stressors like exercise, calorie restriction, low temperature, and oxidative stress, affect mitochondrial biogenesis. Beyond the induction, promotion, stimulation, and inhibition of mitochondrial biogenesis, it is also controlled by other signaling pathways. Not only do differences in mitochondrial mass and number occur during the process, but so do size and mass variations. Research on the regulation of mitochondrial biogenesis is a fast-moving area that has promise for understanding and maybe curing a wide range of human diseases, such as cancer, neurodegenerative diseases, and metabolic disorders.

Research on mitochondrial biogenesis is ongoing and should provide significant new understandings of the function of mitochondria in cellular functions and the consequences of these functions for health and illness. In order to preserve cellular homeostasis and coordinate several cellular processes like energy consumption, cell cycle regulation, and stress responses, mitochondrial biogenesis regulation is a complicated and multifaceted process.

Mitophagy and Autophagy

Two critical processes in the structure and function of mitochondria that are essential to cellular functions are autophagy and mitophagy. Autophagy is a more general process of cellular recycling that gathers cytotoxic senescent organelles and other cellular debris in autophagic vesicles and transports them to lysosomes for destruction. Mitophagy is a selective form of autophagy that involves the degradation of damaged mitochondria.

A crucial quality control system called mitophagy removes damaged mitochondria, stopping the initiation of cell death pathways and guarding against the generation of reactive oxygen species (ROS). The endoplasmic reticulum (ER), mitochondria, and other cellular components can all be specifically targeted by this strictly controlled process. Proteins that modulate mitochondrial dynamics, such as Drp1, which is involved in mitochondrial fission, are in charge of mitophagy.

Conversely, autophagy is a broader process involved in turnover and damage control within cells. It is necessary for preserving cellular homeostasis and is involved in the removal of damaged cellular organelles, including mitochondria. Numerous signaling pathways control autophagy, which can be triggered by a variety of physiological circumstances, including nutrition shortages, aging, and exposure to pollutants in the environment.

For the mitochondria to remain healthy and operate properly, both autophagy and mitophagy are necessary. Numerous illnesses, such as cancer, metabolic problems, and neurological diseases, can result from the dysregulation of these processes. Deciphering the function of mitochondria in cellular activities and their consequences for health and illness requires an understanding of the molecular mechanisms and regulation of mitophagy and autophagy.

Chapter Eight

Emerging Research and Therapeutic Implications

The complex link between mitochondrial dynamics, cellular activities, and disease has been clarified by recent advances in the study of mitochondrial structure and function. Research has demonstrated the importance of mitochondrial structure at different subcellular sizes and how it affects functional trade-offs related to structural changes. One of the most important factors in determining optimal mitochondrial function is the control of the internal morphology of mitochondria, namely the relative size and form of mitochondrial cristae. This control also supports cellular demands. Moreover, a variety of illnesses, such as cancer, metabolic diseases, cardiovascular diseases, and neurodegenerative disorders, have been related to an imbalance in mitochondrial dynamics, highlighting the need to preserve normal mitochondrial function.

The results of this research are also being investigated for their potential therapeutic applications. One such application is to target diseases by modulating mitochondrial dynamics. Furthermore, strategies for assessing modifications in mitochondrial structure and function—particularly in relation to cancer—are being researched in order to pinpoint and detect abnormalities linked to the disease. The vital process by which cells regulate the quantity of mitochondria, known as mitochondrial biogenesis, is also being investigated in relation to a range of disorders, with an emphasis on therapeutic measures to increase mitochondrial biogenesis in order to prevent and treat a variety of maladies.

In general, new studies on the structure and function of mitochondria are offering insightful information on the function of mitochondria in cellular activities and the implications of these findings for both health· and disease. The development of specific therapy techniques to address mitochondrial dysfunction and related disorders is being facilitated by this information.

Mitochondrial Medicine

The study of mitochondrial structure and function in both health and disease is referred to as "mitochondrial medicine," and it focuses on creating novel therapeutic approaches to treat mitochondrial malfunction. The understanding of the role of mitochondria in cellular activities and their implications for a range of diseases, including cancer, neurodegenerative disorders, metabolic problems, and cardiovascular diseases, is causing this discipline to rapidly evolve.

The fundamental function of mitochondria in cellular energy production, metabolism, and signaling has been demonstrated by research in mitochondrial medicine. Numerous human diseases have been connected to mitochondrial malfunction, and there is increasing interest in creating tailored treatment approaches to deal with these disorders. This includes researching the mechanism by which cells make more mitochondria, known as mitochondrial biogenesis, and how it relates to a number of illnesses, including metabolic syndrome, neurodegenerative diseases, and cardiac pathology.

Additionally, the regulation of mitochondrial activity, particularly the study of mitophagy and autophagy, which are critical processes for preserving mitochondrial health and function, has been the focus of recently developed research in mitochondrial medicine. Numerous disorders, including cancer, have these pathways recognized as possible treatment targets. Furthermore, research on mito-nuclear communication—the connection between the cell nucleus and the mitochondria—has shed light on the function of mitochondria in biological processes and the consequences these activities have for both health and sickness.

All things considered, the study of mitochondrial medicine is a dynamic and quickly emerging field of study with significant significance for comprehending the function of mitochondria in biological processes and creating focused therapeutic approaches to treat diseases linked to mitochondrial malfunction.

Targeting Mitochondria for Therapy

One active field of research in mitochondrial medicine involves targeting mitochondria for therapeutic purposes. Numerous human diseases, including cancer, neurological problems, metabolic issues, and cardiovascular diseases, have been related to mitochondrial malfunction.

Consequently, it is essential to find therapeutic approaches to address mitochondrial dysfunction. One method that has been shown to be successful is to target mitochondria using prodrugs or organelle-specific agents. Because mitochondria regulate both apoptosis and the formation of reactive oxygen species (ROS), targeting mitochondria with medicines makes sense from a therapeutic standpoint. Consequently, the foundation for treating a range of disorders may be provided by the targeted delivery of medications to mitochondria.

The crucial process by which cells regulate the quantity of mitochondria, known as mitochondrial biogenesis, is also being investigated in relation to a number of illnesses, with an emphasis on therapeutic measures to increase mitochondrial biogenesis in order to prevent and treat different pathologies. Furthermore, research on autophagy and mitophagy, two vital processes for preserving the health and function of mitochondria, has shed light on the function of mitochondria in cellular processes and the consequences these processes have for both health and disease. Numerous disorders, including cancer, have these mechanisms recognized as possible treatment targets.

Combinatorial vitamin, antioxidant, and co-factor regimens are frequently used as therapeutic interventions for mitochondrial illnesses. These regimens can be further modified in accordance with biochemical reasoning, past experience, and consensus expert opinion. Enhancing optimal enzymatic and cellular performance is the clinical aim of existing medicines, despite the fact that primary mitochondrial dysfunction has no known cure.

For patients with uncommon and severe forms of mitochondrial disease, new treatment options have been found recently.

The development of specific therapeutic techniques to address mitochondrial malfunction and related disorders is being made possible by these developments in mitochondrial medicine.

Future Directions in Mitochondrial Research

Understanding the intricate interactions between mitochondrial structure, function, and cellular activities is the main goal of future approaches in mitochondrial research. Among the important fields of study are:

1. Mitochondrial dynamics: Understanding how mitochondrial structure and function are regulated requires an understanding of mitochondrial dynamics, which includes fission and fusion. The study of the emerging roles of mammalian mitochondrial fission and fusion is centered on the trade-offs that arise from structural changes to the mitochondrion.

2.   Mitochondrial biogenesis: New mitochondria are created from pre-existing ones through the self-renewal process of mitochondrial biogenesis. Understanding the proteins and signaling mechanisms connected to mitochondrial biogenesis has advanced recently. Future studies will concentrate on comprehending the intracellular mechanisms that the key players that drive mitochondrial biogenesis share, as well as the coordination between the nuclear and mitochondrial genomes.

3. Mitochondrial-nuclear communication: Research into the signaling that occurs between the cell nucleus and the mitochondria, or mito-nuclear communication, is now underway. Deciphering the function of mitochondria in cellular activities and their consequences in health and illness requires an understanding of the molecular mechanisms and regulation of mito-nuclear communication.

4. Mitochondrial dysfunction in disease: A variety of human illnesses, including cancer, neurological diseases, metabolic disorders, and cardiovascular diseases, have been related to mitochondrial malfunction. In order to treat mitochondrial dysfunction and the illnesses that accompany it, future research will concentrate on creating focused therapeutic approaches.

5. Mitochondrial medicine: This is a young discipline that aims to treat mitochondrial dysfunction by creating therapeutic interventions and comprehending the role of mitochondria in cellular activities. Subsequent investigations will center on the creation of tailored treatment approaches intended to tackle mitochondrial malfunction and related disorders.

Future directions in mitochondrial research will primarily concentrate on comprehending the intricate interactions that exist between mitochondrial structure, function, and cellular processes. Specifically, these efforts will aim to develop targeted therapeutic approaches that will address mitochondrial dysfunction and the pathologies that are associated with it.

Conclusion

Essential organelles, mitochondria, are involved in metabolism, signaling, and the synthesis of cellular energy. They still have their own circular genome and are encased in a double membrane. Numerous human diseases, including cancer, neurological problems, metabolic issues, and cardiovascular diseases, have been related to mitochondrial malfunction. Consequently, it is essential to find therapeutic approaches to address mitochondrial dysfunction. In order to treat mitochondrial malfunction and the diseases it is linked to, future initiatives in mitochondrial research will concentrate on comprehending the intricate interactions between mitochondrial structure, function, and cellular activities. Understanding the function of mitochondria in cellular processes and their consequences for both health and sickness has been greatly aided by research on mitophagy, autophagy, mito-nuclear communication, and mitochondrial biogenesis. Targeted treatment approaches to treat mitochondrial dysfunction and related disorders are being developed thanks to the growing body of research in mitochondrial medicine.

Summary of Key Concepts

Essential organelles, mitochondria, are involved in metabolism, signaling, and the synthesis of cellular energy. They still have their own circular genome and are encased in a double membrane. Numerous human diseases, including cancer, neurological problems, metabolic issues, and cardiovascular diseases, have been related to mitochondrial malfunction. Consequently, it is essential to find therapeutic approaches to address mitochondrial dysfunction. In order to treat mitochondrial malfunction and the diseases it is linked to, future initiatives in mitochondrial research will concentrate on comprehending the intricate interactions between mitochondrial structure, function, and cellular activities. Understanding the function of mitochondria in cellular processes and their consequences for both health and sickness has been greatly aided by research on mitophagy, autophagy, mito-nuclear communication, and mitochondrial biogenesis. Targeted treatment approaches to treat mitochondrial dysfunction and related disorders are being developed thanks to the growing body of research in mitochondrial medicine.

Implications for Cellular and Medical Research

The importance of mitochondria in cellular functions and their consequences for a range of disorders have been made clear by research on the structure and function of mitochondria. The synthesis of cellular energy, metabolism, and signaling all depend on mitochondria. They still have their own circular genome and are encased in a double membrane. Numerous human diseases, including cancer, neurological problems, metabolic issues, and cardiovascular diseases, have been related to mitochondrial malfunction. Consequently, it is essential to find therapeutic approaches to address mitochondrial dysfunction.

Understanding the intricate interactions between mitochondrial structure, function, and cellular activities is the main goal of future approaches in mitochondrial research. Mitophagy, autophagy, mito-nuclear communication, and mitochondrial biogenesis are important study topics. These procedures have given important new information about the function of mitochondria in cellular functions and the consequences of these functions in health and illness. Targeted treatment approaches to treat mitochondrial dysfunction and related disorders are being developed thanks to the growing body of research in mitochondrial medicine.

In summary, research on the structure and function of mitochondria is crucial because it sheds light on the involvement of mitochondria in cellular activities and the consequences of these processes for both health and sickness. It is anticipated that continued study in this area will result in the creation of focused treatment plans to address diseases related to mitochondrial malfunction and improve patient outcomes across a range of medical problems.

Reference

Alberts, B., Johnson, A., Lewis, J., Raff, M., Roberts, K., & Walter, P. (2002). Mitochondria. NCBI Bookshelf.

Chan, D. C. (2006). Mitochondrial Form and Function. *Annual Review of Cell and Developmental Biology*, 22, 79-99. https://doi.org/10.1146/annurev.cellbio.22.010305.104638

Day, D. A. (2004). Mitochondrial Structure and Function in Plants. In D. A. Day, A. H. Millar, & J. Whelan (Eds.), *Plant Mitochondria: From Genome to Function* (pp. 1-29). Springer. https://doi.org/10.1007/978-1-4020-2400-9_1

DiMauro, S., & Schon, E. A. (Eds.). (2001). Mitochondrial Disorders Caused by Nuclear Genes. Springer.

Palade, G. E. (1967). The Structure of Mitochondria. Academic Press.

Palmeira, C. M., Moreno, A. J., & Madeira, V. M. (Eds.). (2007). Mitochondrial Function: Methods and Protocols. Springer.

Singh, K. K. (Ed.). (2015). Mitochondrial Medicine: Volume I, Probing Mitochondrial Function. Humana Press.

Oliveira, J. M. A., & Esteves, A. R. (Eds.). (2012). Mitochondrial Dysfunction in Neurodegenerative Disorders. Springer.

About Author

Douglas Randall is a medical researcher who has made significant contributions to the field of genetic dysfunction, particularly in the context of mitochondrial health and disease. His work has addressed the genetics of human mental health disorders in model organisms, as well as the epidemiology and treatment of mitochondrial disorders. Randall's research has contributed to the understanding of mitochondrial dysfunction and its implications for various health conditions, including cognitive impairment and metabolic disorders. His work has also involved probing the in vivo dynamics of mitochondria, shedding light on their structural and functional characteristics. Overall, Douglas Randall's research has been instrumental in advancing the knowledge of genetic influences on mitochondrial function and their impact on human health.